Living With Cancer as
"A New Normal"

Living With Cancer as "A New Normal"

◆

A Journey with Cancer through the Eyes of a Caregiver

Dianna Mitchell Marston, Caregiver

iUniverse, Inc.

New York Lincoln Shanghai

Living With Cancer as "A New Normal"
A Journey with Cancer through the Eyes of a Caregiver

Copyright © 2007 by Dianna Marston

iUniverse books may be ordered through booksellers or by contacting:

iUniverse
2021 Pine Lake Road, Suite 100
Lincoln, NE 68512
www.iuniverse.com
1-800-Authors (1-800-288-4677)

Because of the dynamic nature of the Internet, any Web addresses
or links contained in this book may have changed
since publication and may no longer be valid.

This book was written as a source of information through the eyes of a caregiver. The contents of this book are intended to assist caregivers and patients to find a better understanding of cancer and care giving. It offers direction for research, sources for assistance through the medical and insurance communities, where to look for information which pertains to the patient's form of cancer. This book should not be used as a medical guide and all medical needs must be directed to your medical team.

ISBN: 978-0-595-44899-9 (pbk)
ISBN: 978-0-595-89222-8 (ebk)

Printed in the United States of America

I dedicate this book to my husband, Nathan, who passed away May 17, 2002, and to my two daughters, Kaela and Sorrell, who were 14 and 11 when their father was diagnosed with cancer. It is my desire to share what our journey through cancer brought to us as a family. The journey would have been nearly impossible without the wonderful family members and friends who helped and supported us from the moment Nathan was diagnosed with cancer, through his illness and death, and now keep us company as we adjust to our "new normal."

Contents

Acknowledgments

Our love goes to Nathan Burritt Marston who taught us what it takes to grow into a more spiritual human being. He was Nathan, not his cancer. On our journey, he helped us live with life, not death. We learned to love one another from the depth of our souls and to share our lives with total honesty, care, and love. The journey transformed our lives from living on the surface to getting into the depths, meaning, and value of life. To Nathan, who will always be in our hearts.

I especially appreciate my two daughters, Kaela and Sorrell, and all of our family and friends. I would like to thank the health care professionals who gave of themselves through their knowledge and comforted us while we were on our journey. I would like to thank those who listened to us, and who gave so freely of themselves to our family. We appreciate those who donated blood, were tested as potential bone marrow matches, and who donated stem cells for transplant. To those who wrote, sending us their thoughts and love; and those who brought wonderful meals, managed car pools, visited, assisted with home maintenance, and guided us; we send our love. A special thank you goes to all of you who supported our family in a most difficult yet powerful journey. You know who you are and we love you!

A special thanks to Helen Starbuck Pashley, Peter R. Tischler, Marcy Boyle, Frank Mitchell, Gwendolyn Mitchell, Shirley Marston, Leslie Marston, Jeffrey Marston, Maureen Marston, Jill Chamberlin, Susanne Hammond, Deborah Marston, John Harrington, Bradbury Marston, James Murray, Kaela Marston Chaffin, Sorrell Marston, Lorelei Starbuck Sarnella, Justin Chaffin, Susan Kaufman, Randy Kaufman, Alex Mitchell, Elliot Kaufman, Kelly Marston, Emily Marston, Jack Major, Mariann Major, Jack C. Major, Tonya Major, Bob Major, Terrah Major, Ron Keller, Karen Keller, Harry Tolve, Alex Marston, Warren Marston, Dane Murray, Mary Lynn Murray, Sarah Murray,and Penelope Reynolds who offered their help with editing, encouragement, suggestions and endless support throughout this project. I thank you all!

You Can Live With Cancer
as "A New Normal"

Cancer is an emotional word. We all fear the word when we discover a spot or lump on our bodies, feel pain or discomfort and discover the diagnosis is beginning to look like cancer. It catapults into our lives as we begin to experience this serious illness that will require attention. It is the word that leaps to mind when our health care professional makes an immediate opening in their busy schedule to see us and discuss test results.

We first heard the word cancer when my husband and I arrived at our doctor's office and were immediately placed in a consultation room. Hearing the doctor say that my husband had cancer caused our blood to run cold and our bodies to shiver. Fear flashed across our minds and everything from that moment forward seemed to be in a fog. The idea of dealing with cancer itself was new. It raised many questions for us. What did it mean? Where would we go from here? What were the chances of recovery? Suddenly, we found ourselves plunged into a medical maze, wandering from appointment to appointment, all of which seemed so foreign. Medical offices seemed so frightening and sterile. The lives we knew and enjoyed suddenly no longer existed. We had been introduced to our new lives. Our family began to change its needs and priorities. We began looking at life differently and struggled with how to create *Living With Cancer as "A New Normal"*. We found our lives ever changing without any direction in sight.

I wrote this book to help you understand our prospective of *Living With Cancer as "A New Normal"* and our experience which may assist you with your journey after a family member, friend, or even yourself has been diagnosed with cancer. I have written it through my eyes as a caregiver. I have shared my experiences of the journey through my husband's cancer while continuing to raise our children, navigate medical and insurance mazes, and trying to keep life as normal as possible for my family and friends. I offer this book to you as our experience of living as a family and a patient with cancer. It was difficult, sometimes confusing work, living as a family, providing care to Nathan, and keeping our family together as we moved into our "new normal" place in life.

I have designed this workbook to assist you with your cancer journey and offer assistance with a general understanding of steps needed for this journey. Because my experience was that of a caregiver, that is the focus of this book although it should be helpful for cancer patients as well. The workbook lists general questions for you to ask your medical professionals and personnel at your insurance company, employer, Medicare/Medicaid office, disability insurance company, and Social Security office. There are sections for questions and places to record information about medications, legal issues, medical appointments, and organizational tools. I hope to help you understand the journey ahead of you after a diagnosis of cancer by relating our journey and the many effects cancer had on our lives and offer you some assistance along this arduous trek.

Living With Cancer Workbook and Journey

I have designed this workbook to help you keep yourself organized while everything around you seems disorganized and out of sorts. The workbook provides a place for you to record information you will need as you take your steps through the changes you are about to experience. I offer ideas and questions for you to think about, respond to. I have provided checklists to keep track of doctor's appointments, research facilities, laboratories, hospitals, and insurance companies. There are tips and information to help you find your way through the medical world, keep your personal life in order, and keep family and friends informed. I have included directions about where to go for medical needs, financial needs, psychological needs, house and home assistance, and child care assistance. We used this information to reduce our stress, provide information to our health care providers, insurance companies, and disability insurance company, and to simplify our lives.

This workbook illustrates the steps necessary to keep your affairs (e.g., wills, power of attorney, living wills, death certificates) in order and outlines steps to reach healing beyond the disease and find peace within yourself once again. Using the workbook will help you avoid "reinventing the wheel" and thus reduce extra work. You will need to discover your own answers to many of the questions in this workbook; however, this workbook will provide you with options and directions to begin your journey.

Diagnosis

So, a loved one has cancer. What does this really mean to you? How will it affect the patient's life and the lives of those who will be caring for this person?

First, we must focus on what it is you have just heard from health care professionals. In the past, a person diagnosed with cancer was often given a death sentence. This is not always the case now. The medical establishment has made many new advances in the world of oncology (i.e., the study and treatment of cancer and tumors). Many cancers are being treated with a great deal of success and oncologists (i.e., physicians who specialize in cancer diagnosis and treatment) make improvements all the time. A researcher once told me that oncologists must research their cancer specialty approximately four hours per day just to keep up with advances. Research hospitals have employees whose responsibility is to remain up to date with all forms of research including cancer research. Their findings assist doctors with treatment plans and reviewing new trials available to patients, as well as advances in the specialty. Daily we hear through the news media of many advances in the world of cancer, yet this disease still affects many people each year.

Second, cancer is an extremely emotional word that affects our whole life. It is frightening to discover a serious illness which we do not have any experience with or understanding on how to take our next steps. Many of us are never faced with a loved one's diagnosis of cancer. For those of us who are, it is suddenly a frightening reality. When your loved one has been investigated for a lump or an unexplained illness and is given this most unwelcome diagnosis, it creates emotional chaos. Cancer is a word that causes every emotion to flair and everything from that moment forward becomes a fog.

For us, the word cancer was completely unexpected when it became a part of our lives. We have always been health conscious. Annual physicals, healthy foods, exercise, relaxation, spiritual practices, and play time were a part of our everyday lives. We were traveling; Nathan picked up a piece of light weight luggage and felt pain in his back just around his right shoulder blade. It was very painful and unexplainable. When we returned home from our vacation, he visited our primary care doctor. The pain continued to become more intense as the days progressed. Nathan was first given a prescription pain relief medication for about two weeks after seeing our primary care physician. He tried massage therapy, rest and continued to see our primary care physician over the next three months. Nathan had had a complete physical about two months prior to those symptoms and told he was in perfect health, weight was perfect and to continue living exactly as he had been living. Here we were back in visiting his doctor due to this pain in his back. His doctor felt an x-ray was needed to see what was going on inside his body. It discovered the T-6 and T-7 vertebrae had some sort of damage and were showing up as black spots on the x-rays. Additional tests were ordered; blood testing, MRI, CAT scans, etc. Three months after the first symptom was felt in his back, multiple myeloma (a rare form of bone marrow cancer) was discovered and the diagnosis was made.

Our cancer journey had begun. This sudden change took us to a new place in our lives as we discovered *Living With Cancer as "A New Normal"*. Each day was a new discovery for us in this world of cancer. Suddenly, we faced this medical maze and began wandering from appointment to appointment. It all seemed so foreign. Medical offices seemed so frightening and sterile. Our lives did not exist, as we once knew them. Our family began to change its needs and priorities. We began looking at our lives and how we could create a "new normal." We found our lives ever changing without a direction in sight, like driving through a foreign country without a road map.

Your lives may have just changed as well. We listened to our doctors explain what was going on in Nathan's body and the cell changes that were occurring as a result of his diagnosis of multiple myeloma, a rare form of bone marrow cancer. We did not understand most of the information at the beginning because Nathan was a telecommunication analyst and I am an interior designer, far from anything medical. Fortunately, we had several family members and friends in the medical community who were able to translate what we were hearing from our doctors so we could understand it, as well as offer us suggestions about how to educate ourselves further.

Remember, knowledge gives us a sense of power and helps us engage in the healing process. For many people, knowledge is gained through research in medical libraries, on the Internet, from other patients and support groups, from information given to them by doctors, nurses, therapists, nutritionists, and books. Others may gain their knowledge solely through the advice and direction of their medical team. I believe there is only one correct way of gaining knowledge and that is your way. By this, I mean it is your journey, and your family, friends, and medical professionals must honor your choices. It is equally important to honor the feelings of the caregiver and those close to the patient as well.

I also believe we are living until our last breath. I believe those diagnosed with cancer are living with cancer, not dying from it. A patient's positive thought process and surrounding themselves with positive, respectful people allows the person with cancer and their family to remain hopeful. We must remember we are human beings, not a cancer diagnosis. We will all die at some point and a diagnosis of cancer is not always a death sentence. It is just a diagnosis of a disease with which we must deal and it can be a wake-up call to healthy living and reprioritizing our lives.

There are many theories about the causes of cancer. Many people believe that it is a result of "dis-ease" of the body, mind, and spirit. Some believe cancer is a dysfunction of one's genetic structure. Others think an exposure to cancer-causing agents is the cause. Poor nutrition is believed by some to be the cause of healthy cells becoming cancerous. Research has shown that some cancers originate from viral infection. Whatever the cause or the triggering factor that resulted in healthy cells becoming cancerous, the fact is when cancer is present we must take steps to heal.

There are many cancer treatment choices today. All choices have their own risks and benefits. Patients must choose a treatment direction that serves them best. It is important for patients to examine their belief structure, emotions, and review what is important to them personally.

Always remember everyone; including those in the medical profession, think their way is the best and healthiest way to treat cancer. We found believing in our team of health care professionals was important. Our team consisted of a number of people and began first with Nathan at the helm. We began with our primary care physician, who referred us to a back specialist, an orthopedic (bone) specialist, a general oncologist, a hematology oncologist (a specialist in cancers of the blood and bone marrow), a neurological (brain) specialist, a radiation (x-ray) specialist, and a bone marrow specialist. We also saw magnetic resonance imaging (MRI) staff, a computed axial tomography (CAT) scan specialist, and members of the bone marrow transplant team. As you can see, we had quite a number of people on our medical team. We put together a team that supported us and included a research support group specializing in multiple myeloma that taught us about this form of bone marrow cancer. We met with a nutritionist to support Nathan's immune system. A hypnotherapist taught us how to deal with our stress and help us focus on healing the "dis-ease" in Nathan's body. Physical and Occupational Therapists helped Nathan adjust to the changes within his body and his ability to function in his daily life. We met with doctors all over the world specializing in multiple myeloma. We also brought together family and friends who helped us with our personal lives.

We spent many long hours in clinics, hospitals, and at appointments. My days as a caregiver often lasted 18 hours or more per day and this went on for months. Family and friends offered support in many ways. They raised money so we were able to travel to a multiple myeloma specialist in Germany. Meals were brought to us regularly to relieve us from the responsibility of grocery shopping and cooking. They placed their home-cooked meals in an ice chest next to our door for months. Friends organized car pools and drove our children to and from school and activities. They created a community of love and attention for our children as Nathan and I moved into our new normal and through the treatment process. Many family and friends came from other parts of the country to stay with us and helped with house cleaning, yard care, and laundry, cooking and shopping, and helped us simply keep our lives afloat. We notified teachers of Nathan's illness, and many kept our daughters after school to assist them with their homework and were available to listen to anything they wanted to talk about.

We spent many days driving hundreds of miles from specialist to specialist, to treatments, to hospitals, and back home. I found those days in the car very fatiguing. It seemed as if I listened to every radio station and every song ever played on the air. I listened to my CDs so often I knew the lyrics by heart. I found renting books on CD was a lifesaver. Books on CDs brought me a great deal of peace, escape from life's issues, and gave me something fresh to think about. I would drive and listen to the book. It took my mind off Nathan's illness and helped me actually look forward to driving. At times, I could not wait to jump in the car, drive for an hour, and listen to my book.

TIP

Remember, on top of your new responsibilities, life continues as it normally does when a loved one has cancer. Many caregivers continue with full-time jobs, family and home responsibilities, and other activities. Look for assistance wherever it is available. Consider alternative ways of working—telecommuting or taking a leave of absence. Some states are currently offering financial assistance to caregivers. Check with your state government to see if you qualify for assistance. Look into hiring or asking a friend to help with home maintenance. Allow others to step in and help where they can. People enjoy helping others and it allows them to feel like they are a part of the healing process.

Part of my healing process began by closing my business and enjoying every minute we had together as a family. I knew deep within me I needed to do everything possible to give Nathan his best chance for life and help him experience each day at its very best. My daughters and I wanted his life to be as comfortable as it could be. Our daughters were very much a part of Nathan's treatment plan and this brought a new closeness to our family that seemed to help our daughters feel safe. Nathan and I listened to their thoughts and emotions, and we considered their ideas regarding treatment choices and the direction we were going. During Nathan's illness, we worked on projects, played games, watched movies, talked, and worked on homework as a family. This gave our daughters and me a great deal of comfort as we processed Nathan's death and "living yet another new normal" after this journey of his cancer.

Nathan was our daughters' soccer coach as well as their dad. He coached both daughters from early elementary school until he was hospitalized. We found that taping their games while Nathan was in the hospital helped him feel a part of our daughters' lives. We taped games, brought them to the hospital, and watched them together as a family. The team members and their parents would tape messages to Nathan after each game for him to watch and listen to. Nathan would offer coaching advice to the kids and the new coach. These helped the team play, reach a "new normal" and still enjoy Nathan's presence. Nathan and I tried to maintain a normal life, build memories for our daughters, and help all of us feel as if we were living a normal life as much as possible. This all gave us a message that life had not stopped, and created many loving, fun family memories.

Support Groups:
Help Along the Way

The cancer journey is a bumpy ride; the road is unclear; there are no directions, and sometimes life feels like a roller coaster. Support groups are a huge help. Talking with people who are experiencing some of the same things you are is crucial. They can help you understand what is happening, offer different points of view, provide information to which you may not have access to, and alert you to potential problems. Most importantly, they can give you truly empathetic support when you need it, which others, who have not shared the cancer journey experience, cannot.

Our North Texas Myeloma Support Group was a lifesaver as far as I am concerned. Every patient in this group had multiple myeloma (MM) and everyone without MM was a caregiver. Each of us had an important role in this group. Amazingly enough, we each brought our specialty to our meetings. Some people were members of the health care community—doctors, nurses, and psychologists. Members outside the medical community had computer knowledge, accounting skills, and the ability to write a newsletter. We all had one thing in common and that was MM. Each person had his or her own amazing story to tell, which helped other members live in a positive healthy way while *Living With Cancer as "A New Normal"*. The group offered education, an emotional pillar, friendships, and availability for whoever needed assistance, guidance, or support. Our support group held me together during Nathan's illness and helped me tremendously after his death. When you are dealing with cancer, you need support. Those who are having similar experiences are able to truly understand your feelings, emotions, and needs.

Finding the right support group is important and is a very personal choice. Peter (patient) and Lucy (caregiver) founded our MM support group and came to our home just after Nathan was diagnosed. They talked to us in a very positive way. They explained the disease, talked about the support group, answered our questions, and gave us a direction to take as we began our journey. The MM group met monthly to discuss each person's experiences with treatments, new treatment options just being released from trial stages, available medications—how they worked and their side effects, offered guidance about helping patients and their families with assistance programs available to both patients and caregivers. Marsha (a caregiver) was indispensable when Nathan was critically ill, by connecting us to doctors who provided additional cutting-edge medical treatment through a world renowned specialist who improved his condition. She talked to me about his condition, lent her ears and shoulders to me when I needed to release concerns, feelings and emotions, guided me to the people with specific expertise needed, and held me together emotionally during this entire process. We developed a friendship that lasts to this day.

It is very important to find people who can offer you support, understanding, and guidance when you need it, and who can help you find a direction that serves you best. You can find wonderful specialty cancer support groups as well as many general cancer support groups. Many people find it helpful to belong to both types of groups. It, of course, depends on you and your needs. We found our specialty group through a friend who was dealing with cancer and his friend had multiple myeloma (the exact form of cancer as Nathan's diagnosis). Ask people you meet at the hospital treatment center or someone you know who has cancer if they belong to a support group and what their thoughts are about their group.

TIP

Talk to your medical professionals about a support group for your type of cancer. Contact hospitals, churches, and The American Cancer Society for listings of groups in your area. Use the Internet to locate groups in your area and those specializing in your type of cancer.

There are several things to keep in mind when searching for a group. The Internet offers many sites to visit. Not all sites have scientific backing or are as reliable as other sites. We found it important to take the information we found on the Internet, books and any other forms of information to our doctors and support group for their opinion. As you search for a group, remember that a group is only what its members make it, so finding the right one for you may take visiting a few groups. Sometimes, revisiting a group later will help you find one that best fits your needs.

Regardless of what you learn or discuss in a support group, it is important to follow your oncologist's treatment plan and ask to review your discoveries before you decide to act on anything. Our doctors learned a lot about different treatments available around the world through our research. Some treatments they agreed with and others they did not. It is important to discuss anything you find that is of interest to you with your medical team. Never take or try something you find on the Internet or from any other source before you know exactly how it works, its reliability and side effects, and how it may possibly interfere with your current treatment. Always talk to your medical team before taking anything internally or applying it to your body. Adverse effects may occur that complicate your treatment and recovery.

We found the following sites to be reliable. Often they directed us to other sites for further research.

American Cancer Society

www.cancer.org
1-800-ACS-2345

MD Anderson Hospital

www.mdanderson.org
1-800-393-1611 option 3 to speak to a person

National Cancer Institute—Cancer Information Center

Bethesda, MD 20892
www.ncinih.gov/clinicaltrials
1-800-422-6237

City of Hope

Southern California biomedical research and treatment center, and hospital for cancer
www.cityofhope.org
1-877-482(hope) 4673
City of Hope National Medical Center
1500 E. Duarte Road, Duarte, CA 91010

National Coalition for Cancer Survivorship

www.canceradvocacy.org
1-888-650-9127
To find other research-oriented institutions: www.cancer.org/asp/search/ftc/ftc_global.asp

After Diagnosis:
Developing Your Travel Plan

Once someone has experienced the shock of a diagnosis of cancer, time is needed to rest and to understand what this diagnosis really means. As our fog of diagnosis cleared we had a challenge awaiting us. This is where this workbook will come in handy.

In all probability, you will meet with your medical professionals after the initial diagnosis to gain a better understanding of the disease and what it means to you personally. Bring your workbook and take notes. Any diagnosis, but especially cancer and the fear and confusion it engenders, can cause people to forget what their physician may tell them. The first part of your workbook deals with the first few appointments after diagnosis and gives you space to take notes. This information will be helpful to have and review at home when you have time. I guarantee you will not remember many of the things spoken to you by the time you return home unless you are a medical person—and sometimes not even then! This information will also help you when seeing other healthcare providers or on admission to a hospital and make these experiences much less stressful.

The workbook is a good place to record information which may be needed later and which may be required by caregivers other than your primary care provider or oncologist. Some of the crucial pieces of information include

- Type of cancer. There are many forms of cancer. You need to know the kind of cancer you are dealing with and how it affects the human body.

- The stage. Cancer is rated by stages and the stage of your cancer will help determine a treatment plan. Staging is also used with health insurance to determine how your health insurance will be processed.

- Prognosis. Prognosis is important as it affects the choices for treatment plans as well as expectations for each treatment.

- Treatment options. These vary depending on the cancer you have and the stage at which it has been diagnosed. Treatment options also change based on a patient's response.

Ask as many questions as you can so you will have a better understanding of what to expect during treatment. If necessary, write down your own questions in this book or add additional paper to record your questions and leave space for the response. Also, ask about treatments that are being researched and are in clinical trials. If you choose to participate in a clinical trial, will that interfere with current treatment or keep you from getting another form of treatment in the future? Many of the drugs and protocols used to treat cancer are toxic to various body systems and may have lifetime toxicity levels. The drugs used to treat cancer are often part of a protocol which research has shown to be successful. Their effects on body systems may mean that they cannot be used repeatedly. The consequences of treatment protocols must be explained before administration so that you are giving informed consent. This may mean that a physician explains this to you in language that he or she understands and which is not clear to you. It is your responsibility to ask questions until it makes sense to you.

Reading about Nathan's multiple myeloma helped us understand treatment plans, the doctor's terminology, test results, and a holistic approach to cancer. We discovered we had a responsibility as a patient and caregiver to help with the healing process. We also discovered it is very important to research the information we were receiving. There is a lot of information found on the Internet, in books and in magazines that is not correct. You must be careful about your sources. We found research libraries at the cancer hospitals to be a very good source of information as well as information from the National Institutes of Health.

The Internet, books, and magazines can all provide excellent information as long as you can verify two things: one, where it originated and two, the credentials of those providing the information. You will find information on conventional treatments, alternative treatments, complementary treatments, and information to help support body systems while going through treatment. Ask your medical team for Internet sites, books, and magazines for you to read so you can educate yourselves with the form of cancer with which you are dealing with. We found additional direction for our personal research through web sites, books and magazines given to us by our medical team. It is also very important to understand the medications the patient is taking and what the effects may have on their body while in treatment and afterwards. Research on your part will help you determine the kind of treatment which best accommodates your belief system, the treatment options available, what you or your insurance will pay for, and how to find free or low-cost treatments that may be available.

TIP

Ask your doctors and nurses for copies of your test results.
Ask them to explain what the test results mean.

Healthcare providers are happy to share this information with you. We found the numbers on the laboratory work to be a blur when discussed in the doctor's office. Taking the test results home and reading them helped us to process the information, treatments, and planning, which, in turn, helped relieve stress. Some of the laboratory results may be confusing or look out of line when reading the reports. Remember, only your doctor can translate this information in a meaningful way.

We found keeping a notebook with this information was most important. It helped us remember information when seeing a new doctor or referred to a specialist. Many times your oncologist will request a visit with another doctor or specialist to review your case. It is much easier to have reports regarding this information (blood work, CAT scans, MRIs, X-rays) available in a notebook that you can take with you to avoid delays, confusion, and frustration, than to totally rely on hospitals and offices to forward information. We also kept notes from each doctor's visit to help explain why we were visiting the next specialist. Many times it is helpful to electronically record your doctor visits, if your doctor gives permission to do so. Some appointments offer so much information it is difficult to write all of the information down at the appointment and understand it when you return home. Also, we found recording the appointment allowed us to listen, form questions and understand the information being given at the time of the appointment. It gave us a way to refer back to information which seemed unclear once we arrived home. Keeping a notebook like this will allow quick access to your records. It is a lot of extra work for you as a patient or caregiver to gather this information if you must go to each office and request your files to take with you to a new appointment or hospital visit. We carried our notebook even when we traveled on vacations. It was quite useful when Nathan needed medical attention while away from home. We could show a new doctor all of Nathan's medications, treatments, past tests—all the information a new doctor might need to treat Nathan.

Our notebook was a lifesaver when Nathan required two bone marrow transplants. We had to move from one hospital to another with an entirely new medical team. We were able to refer to our notebook and show the doctors who he had seen, what treatments he had received, and all medical procedures he had undergone without missing a single important piece of information. The transplant team was able to contact each medical facility and request any additional records needed. We were not stressed trying to remember what had happened when, and who had participated in the treatment. We were able to use our time to follow up with Nathan's siblings who were potential stem cell donors. Once the perfect match with Nathan's brother Jeff was in place, we began another section in our notebook. We placed all of the necessary information about the potential transplant in our notebook—transplant options, potential donors names, preparations required for the transplant, and tests required for transplant.

As you can see, your notebook will grow in the direction your treatment takes. Each notebook is individual and personal to each patient. Remember that cancer treatment should care for the whole patient—nutrition, spiritual aspects, mental attitude, and physical illness. Hospitals, doctors, and support groups can refer you to resources that help the patient and the caregiver fight the cancer physically, mentally, and spiritually.

TIP

Your notebook is a good place to keep a list of all the medications that the patient is currently taking and the side effects they cause. This will help identify the source of problems if they occur.

Cancer patients go through a tremendous amount of discomfort because of the medications and treatments used. Medications given to treat cancer, like any other medication, cause changes within the body in addition to the effects for which they are given. This can mean changes in mood or personality that make the patient appear unlike himself or difficult to deal with. Remember to talk to your doctor if you see changes such as these and ask for assistance with dealing with them. Find out what the side effects of each medication are and how they affect the individual. For example, steroids, which are commonly used during chemotherapy, may cause patients to become agitated, angry, upset, or unable to sleep, and generally cause one to become ravenous. An angry, irritable, insomniac loved one can stress even the most loving relationship to its limit. Try to remember, it is the disease and medication talking, not your loved one.

Where possible, seek help to counteract the side effect that is altering the patient's health and quality of life. As the caregiver, you may notice these changes much faster than your medical team. There is never a stupid question and anything you believe is not normal needs to be brought to your medical team's attention. Emergencies can arise while under treatment. Some side effects that require quick medical attention include

- elevated body temperature,

- abdominal bloating,

- changes in pain level and discomfort,

- vomiting, and

- blood pressure changes.

- abnormal breathing patterns

It is important to ask your health care providers for symptoms you should watch for during each phase of treatment and during the relatively normal times between treatments. At one point, Nathan was on steroids that caused his blood sugar to rise. Our physician told us to watch for dryness in the mouth, visual changes, and mood alterations. We noticed some of these changes and contacted our doctors. A simple blood sugar test revealed that he had become diabetic while on this medication. His blood sugar level was high enough to cause a diabetic coma and he had to be hospitalized and treated. He was well after two days when his blood sugar stabilized. It was the dryness in his mouth and the visual change that alerted us to the need for care. Had our physician not warned us to look for this, we might not have noticed until he was gravely ill. We kept in close contact with all of our medical team and you will find a form in your workbook to record who you should contact at any given time.

TIP

**Remember to take your medical notebook to emergency room
visits to assist staff members in providing the best medical
care for your loved one.**

Remember, emergencies do arise as many changes occur within the body. When dealing with an emergency, it is important to tell the hospital staff that the patient has cancer and is on immunosuppressant medications. When a person's immune system is suppressed, it cannot protect the individual from infection as it should. It is important for them to stay away from sick people, as much as possible. On arrival at the emergency room, alert the staff to your condition and ask to go through triage and be placed in a room away from the waiting area to reduce your exposure to illnesses.

It is advisable for cancer patients to protect themselves from germs when in public. This includes thorough, frequent hand washing, use of masks to prevent respiratory illnesses; use of gloves or disposable towels to open doors or when touching other public surfaces, and requiring people around the cancer patient to be healthy and up on their vaccinations. It is a much healthier practice to learn how to prevent the spread of illnesses by following your health care provider's guidelines and the tips mentioned above.

Additional web sites you may want to research:
Mayo Clinic Cancer Centers

www.cancercenter.mayo.edu
www.mayoclinic.com/health/cancer
www.mayoclinic.org
Jacksonville (904) 953-2000
Rochester (507) 284-2511
Arizona (480) 301-8000

University of Arkansas for Medical Sciences

www.uams.edu
1-800-942-8267.
4301 W. Markham St., Little Rock, AR 72205
To make an appointment call The Appointments Center at 1-501-686-8000 or
For general information and for numbers not listed, call 1-501-686-7000

City of Hope Cancer Center

General information about City of Hope
www.cityofhope.org
622-256-HOPE (4673) Information Packet request form

University of Colorado Health Sciences Center—Dennison Library

www.uccc.info
4200 E. 9th Ave. A003
Denver, CO 80262-0003
303-315-7460
Access to its contents is on PubMed if you can't actually physically visit.

Sidney Kimmel Comprehensive Cancer Center at Johns Hopkins

www.hopkinskimmelcancercenter.org
Main telephone 410-955-5000

Kimmel Cancer Center

www.hopkinskimmelcancercenter.org
410-955-5222
401 North Broadway
Baltimore, MD 21231

Dana-Farber Cancer Institute Boston

http://dana-farber.org
617-632-3000
44 Binney Street
Boston, MA 02115

Massachusetts General Hospital Cancer Center

www.massgeneral.org
1-877-726-5130 or 617-726-5130
55 Fruit Street
Boston, MA 02114

Memorial Sloan-Kettering Cancer Center

www.mskcc.org
212-639-2000
1275 York Avenue
New York, NY 10021

Baylor University Medical Center

www.bhcs.com
1800-4BAYLOR (1-800-422-9567)
3490 Worth Street
Sammons Tower
Dallas, TX 75246

University of Texas M.D. Anderson Cancer Center

www.mdanderson.org
1-800-392-1611 or 1-713-792-6161
1515 Holcombe Blvd.
Houston, TX 78030

University of Washington Medical Center

www.uwmedicine.org
206-598-3300
1959 NE Pacific
Seattle, WA 98195

Fred Hutchinson Cancer Research Center

www.fhcrc.org
206-667-5000
1100 Fairview Ave. North
Seattle, WA 98019

University of Wisconsin Comprehensive Cancer Center

www.cancer.wisc.edu
800-622-8922
600 Highland Ave
Madison, WI 53792

Clinical Trials Information:
Thomson Centerwatch Clinical Trials Listing Service

www.centerwatch.com
(617) 856-5900
Call for oncology clinical trials. You can search for investigational studies.

National Cancer Institute's Cancer Information Service

www.nci.nih.gov/clinicaltrials
(800) 422-6237

National Cancer Institute's Clinical Studies Support Center

www.ccr.ncifcrf.gov/trails/cssc
(888) 624-1937
Clinical Trials with your type and stage of cancer

Home In A New Light

Home preparation is imperative when you have a cancer patient taking medications, balance issues, physical changes which take place during treatments and finding that new normal place within their home. Germ control during treatment, preventing falls, access to the kitchen, bathrooms, bedrooms, living areas are all a large part of *Living With Cancer as "A New Normal"*.

We were given information by our medical staff and found through our research how to prepare our home for protecting as much as possible against transmitting germs among each other, preventing falls, access to all parts of our home, lighting and even sound so that we were able to make our home as comfortable as possible for Nathan.

Germs are a major issue when a cancer patient is on treatment and their immune system is compromised (unable to fend off infections). Healthy people and cleanliness does not just happen. It is something we all must think about. People who are close to and caring for the cancer patient must try to stay healthy so that the patient does not become ill by our passing of germs. Of course, we all have times of illness and must be near the patient. We were given information which helped us stay healthy and when we were not feeling well, we were able to keep as many germs away from Nathan as possible by taking a few precautions.

Washing of hands is one of the most important factors of keeping germs under control. Always cover ones mouth when sneezing and coughing with a disposable tissue and wash hands well with soap and water. When ill, use surgical gloves and masks when near patient. We tried to stay away from unhealthy people as much as possible so that we did not become ill and bring those germs back to our home. Ask your health care providers for additional health suggestions and tips.

The kitchen was cleaned with vinegar or bleach water by washing the sink, faucets, counter tops, door handles/pulls, oven handles, refrigerator handles, dishwasher, garbage disposal, etc. after each use. Most home dishwashers do not reach a high enough water temperature to kill all germs and bacteria which can be left behind on "clean" dishes and spread viruses.

Tip

Pour a cup of vinegar in the bottom of the empty dishwasher and run it through the normal wash cycle about every third load. This helps to prevent many germs and bacteria from building up inside of your dishwasher.

It is important to wash door knobs off daily with vinegar or a bleach water solution to keep as clean as possible. Bathrooms should be cleaned daily with the same care as in the kitchen. Wash the sinks, faucets, toilets, tubs and showers after each use or designate one bathroom to be the cancer patient's bathroom. Computer keyboards collect many germs from the family. A patient may want to wear a light weight surgical glove when using the computer. Telephones are also great germ collectors so remember to wipe them down daily as well.

Accessibility for people now using additional equipment to stay mobile (walkers, canes, wheelchairs) sometimes requires a few changes to be made around the house. Guard rails may need to be installed on both sides of the stair cases, grips installed on the walls in the showers and bath tubs, near toilets, higher toilet seats attached to the toilets, wider door openings for wheel chairs, flooring changes to keep floors level without area rugs to trip over, changing the kitchen storage around for lower access and many other items can be changed to fit the needs for each individual. Many times changes are temporary and other times changes are permanent depending on the cancer and the patient's needs.

Safety is the most important factor to consider when thinking of making changes. Nathan would seem to be stable on his feet and raise one foot to step into the shower, lose his balance and fall to the floor. It was so important for someone to be with him that was strong enough to keep him from falling. Falling happens and when it does it can be very serious. So remember to keep floors free of clutter, remove sharp edged furniture from your home or covered with child guard protectors, cover tile floors in bathrooms with slip resistant rugs and reduce the number of obstacles.

Furniture arrangements and room traffic patterns can help a person's ability to access a room comfortably and limit falls. Take a moment in each room and determine how that room is used and walk through the room using a walker to see if the room allows ease of moment and is safe for each person to use. It is important for the caregiver to try using a walker, wheel chair or cane in each room of the house to see where obstacles may be located and correct traffic patterns as needed. Experiencing accessibility issues also offers the caregiver a better understanding of the patients needs and can help prevent serious injuries down the road. A safe home is a happy home!

Tip

Ask for assistance from your health care professionals, interior designers and social workers for preparing your home for this new health condition. Many homes are accidents waiting to happen for people who have balance issues and need grips in showers, extra guard rails near stairs, changes in flooring to help the patient walk and use walkers, wheel chairs, kitchen accessibility, beds, chairs, etc.

Some treatments cause a cancer patient to lose their ability to be able to see well in low lighting. Lighting in your home is very important for safety reasons and can be dealt with easily. Brighter lights can be purchased through department stores and lighting stores for very reasonable prices. Many people have added directional floor lamps (pole lights with flexible or hinged adjustable lights) so that shadows are not present. Think of driving on a very sunny day and now entering a tunnel, then exiting the tunnel in bright sun again. For a moment it is difficult for our eyes to adjust to the light changes. A cancer patient may have this kind of dramatic change just moving around in a room with slight shadows and back to a low light area. The lighting can be dramatic and needs to be considered to keep accidents from happening.

Keeping Others Healthy Around The Cancer Patient

Our family had children in school during Nathan's time with cancer. Our older child was in 9th grade and mostly free of childhood illnesses. Our younger child was in 6th grade in the middle of childhood illnesses. We worked very hard on keeping our family healthy during treatment times as well as healthy times. It was difficult, but we managed.

We found keeping up with recommend vaccinations kept us all healthy. Sometimes we forget that boosters are necessary later in life to keep childhood illnesses under control.

Tip

Check with your medical office to see if every member of your family's vaccinations is up to date. Keep in mind those booster shots for vaccinations we received as children are necessary later in life. Your doctor will be able to give you all of the information you need to keep up to date with your vaccinations.

We also were told by a member of the medical community how important it is to keep up on nutrition and how nutrition is the first line of defense of illness. We visited with a nutritionist who recommend a general meal plan to help us keep our meals well balanced, organic (keeping excess chemicals away from our daily food intake), suggested healthy snack foods and staying away from fast foods as much as possible. We began taking a supplement called "Juice Plus" which helped all of us stay healthy during a time when a meal schedule was next to impossible. We made a shake, took our supplements, packed healthy lunches in the morning before our children were sent off to school and we were off to Nathan's treatments. We always ate healthy foods but found that we needed some changes to our diets after talking to our nutritionist. Once we began making those changes and taking "Juice Plus", we found ourselves with fewer viruses, bacterial infections and in general, in better health. Needless to say our worries of dealing with childhood illnesses and pesky viruses began to disappear simply by treating ourselves to healthier meals, supplements, resting as much as possible and taking stress free moments for ourselves.

Tip

Ask your health care professional for suggestions to help your family stay healthy. Ask questions about products such as "Juice Plus" and other supplements which may help you prevent illnesses, amount of exercise, how often, number of hours of rest and general health questions suited to meet your family needs. Remember how important it is for the caregiver to remain healthy and protect yourselves during this major change in your life.

Transplant and Donation:
A Gift of Life

We hear about transplants in the news and other media, as well as from the medical community. Transplants are accomplished when another living person shares an organ or part of one, or provides stem cells or bone marrow to another person. Organs also can be transplanted from people who have died and have previously arranged for donation of their organs. It is truly the gift of life. I like to think of a transplant as a gift given by a person to improve the quality of life for someone else. It is also a gift of life from a deceased person who arranges to share his or her organs, as a piece of them is still living.

In an attempt to kill the multiple myeloma cancer cells produced in his bone marrow, Nathan's bone marrow needed to be destroyed by chemotherapy and radiation. To survive this, Nathan required a bone marrow transplant. This was first accomplished using stem cells harvested from Nathan himself at a time when his cancer was in remission. This is called an autologous transplant, meaning the stem cells come from the patient receiving it. In other words, you donate to yourself. Physicians removed stem cells from his blood and stored them in liquid nitrogen at the hospital for future use. He donated his cells about one year into his treatment and used them four years later. It provided a good bridge and gave us time to consider other options. His physicians hoped that this bone marrow did not contain cancer cells because he was in remission. He received the stem cells after chemotherapy and radiation treatment that prepared him for the transplant. This treatment put Nathan into another remission. Nathan's remission was intended to give his body the time to enable him to properly receive his brother's stem cells in a second transplant. This meant that Jeff (Nathan's brother) became the stem cell donor and the source of healthy bone marrow stem cells to use for transplant in the hopes that Nathan would go in to a longer or possibly permanent remission. This is known as a heterologous or allogeneic transplant and means that the tissue comes from another person or source.

We began the process by trying to find someone who was as close a genetic match as possible to Nathan. This is done by testing blood for all of the transplant match markers. Normally, the search begins by testing family members, as it is more likely that a good match will be found there. Nathan has siblings. His two sisters were close matches to Nathan, but his brother Jeff was the best match. Jeff, Deborah, and Leslie all wanted to offer Nathan another chance at a complete healing. Jeff was chosen because his stem cells were the closest match. Jeff completed his physical examination and began preparing to donate his stem cells to his brother. Before the harvest, he was given a medication that caused his bone marrow to produce more stem cells than his body needed. He then began the aphaeresis or harvesting process, a three-hour procedure that removes blood from one of the donor's arms, separates out the stem cells, and returns the rest of the blood to the donor's other arm. The harvested stem cells were stored in a blood transfusion bag, from which the cells were transferred to Nathan similar to a blood transfusion.

Many times a perfect match is not found within the family members. There are transplant banks where people are tested for transplant donations and their information is stored on a computer program. Once the family can not donate to the patient the transplant banks are notified. The patient's transplant match markers are entered into a computer search for a donor whose transplant match markers match the patient's markers. Additional testing is then performed on those who match the first search until a donor is found.

The entire procedure is a miracle and such a gift of life. New transplant advances are discovered each day and affect patients everywhere. Organ donation is something that is very personal and should be carefully considered by each person. Please consider giving to another person, if asked, and talk to your doctor for advice when considering this gift. If you choose to donate organs after death, you can indicate this in many states on your driver's license. You may want to indicate this in your medical power of attorney forms or living will. You should discuss your requests and decisions with family members so that they are informed and in agreement with you as they will be making decisions for you, should you need them to make arrangements for you.

It is also important to remember how important it is to donate blood products. All cities have collection centers and are always in need of blood products to give to cancer patients as well as patients with other illnesses and injuries. A cancer patient may require platelets, plasma, and whole blood transfusions, all of which require many donors. We need to keep blood products available to patients in need, and donating blood is very simple. Please consider the gift of life by donating blood products on a regular basis. You are the one who can save another person's life and offer them healing.

Notebook Shopping List

I highly recommend keeping Medical and Insurance Notebooks as well as this workbook. The workbook will provide information needed regularly with names, phone numbers, addresses, and directions. The Medical Notebook will assist the caregiver with filing and organizing all the patient records of medical treatments, test results, medications, and other information. The Insurance Notebook will help keep track of expenses, co-pays, covered by insurance or patient responsibility statements.

Here is a general list of supplies for the Medical Notebook. If you need records that are more detailed, you can purchase additional dividers and labels to customize the Medical Notebooks. All supplies can be purchased at any store with office supplies.

It is helpful for you to purchase the following for your <u>Medical Notebook</u>:

- One three-ring binder to keep track of your records,

- Two packages of three-ring binder tabs,

- Two packages of three-ring binder pockets,

- One package of three-ring binder business card plastic pockets, and

- A daily planner or calendar to record all of your appointments (you can find a three ring binder planner that can be fastened in your notebook).

It is helpful to purchase the following for your <u>Insurance Notebook:</u>

- One three-ring binder to keep track of your records,

- Two packages of three-ring binder tabs,

- Two packages of three-ring binder pockets, and

- One package of three-ring binder business card plastic pockets

Medical and Insurance Notebooks

We used a three-ring binder for each notebook to keep track of records, two packages of three ring binder tabs to organize records within the binder, and one package of three ring binder pockets which allowed a pocket to hold information gathered at each appointment until we were home and able to place it behind the correct tab. We used one package of three ring binder business card plastic pockets for keeping track of phone numbers and addresses for each healthcare provider. Our doctors loved the notebook because it took all of the guesswork out of translating from our language into medical terms.

Create two three-ring binder notebooks, titled Medical and Insurance: We used the following headings for each divider; you may come up with different ones that are more helpful to you.

Doctors Visits. We filed these by date of service. It can be helpful if you create a tab for each doctor or medical person you see regularly. You can file all future information from that person in the appropriate section.

Laboratory Results. We filed these by date of test and included the test results.

Other tests. MRI, CAT scans, etc.

Prescriptions/medications prescribed by your doctors. It is helpful to keep track of these for reference.

Hospital reports and visits. Having a record of all visits and other information pertaining to the visits is helpful especially when providing a new health care provider with a history of treatment.

Emergency Room visits. Information about any ER visits will help your health care providers stay up to date on your treatment. ERs do not always reliably send information to the primary care provider or oncologist after an ER visit.

Medical Insurance:
The Fuel For Your Journey

Medical care, especially for cancer, is costly. Many people have medical insurance, but coverage for prescriptions and medical care (especially specialty care that is needed to treat cancer) varies from policy to policy. I found the best way to learn what the patient's insurance policy will cover was simply to call the telephone number on their insurance card. It is helpful for both patient and caregiver to read the patient policy handbook to become familiar with what is covered and what is not. Information given over the phone may be confusing or inaccurate. If the patient and caregiver are familiar with the patient policy handbook, one can ask informed questions. It is always wise when speaking over the phone to a representative, to record the date, the person's name with whom you are speaking, and a phone number. You, unfortunately, may have to refer to this later.

The patient's workbook provides space to document this information while on the phone with the patient's insurance carrier. Ask to speak to an insurance representative, who can explain:

- how this policy functions

- what its limitations are

- how the referral process works

- the policy benefits

The representative can explain how to file a claim. Depending on the patients policy, claims may be filed by the patient or caregiver after the patient has received a service or most often they will be filed directly by the medical providers. Ask the representative to explain the following:

- plan co-pays and deductibles

- length of time to receive reimbursements

- coverage for drug or treatment trials

- caps for the plan (many insurance plans have a lifetime coverage limit)

- what is required from you to be covered by the plan, receive medical care and payments

- the availability of a person to handle your case on a continuing basis

It is very important to know this information as soon as the diagnosis has taken place.

Most insurance companies have a person who will work with the patient and caregiver on a continuing basis in the claims department. Calling the insurance company at the time of diagnosis is important. It informs them that a diagnosis of cancer has been made and gives the patient and caregiver an opportunity to ask for help processing claims. They can also share with you services that are available to patients with long term illnesses. My husband's account was assigned to a caseworker who helped us process the claims, which were processed in Texas and paid through Chicago. Our claims totaled approximately one million dollars. To avoid reaching the allowable lifetime cap, you may need to ask the insurance company not to pay certain charges that you could pay for out of pocket. This is yet another reason to keep up with insurance claims. If the patient is nearing the cap on their policy, one can make informed decisions about what charges to submit to the insurance company and what to pay for themselves.

It is helpful to create a notebook titled "Insurance" where both patient and caregiver can file the doctor's charges for each visit by dates of service. This helps ease the confusion of dealing with the insurance company and the billing received from health care providers after a service has occurred. Often, you may not know the doctors who are billing the insurance company such as for radiology or anesthesia services. Often, the patient or caregiver will receive information from their insurance company telling them they are paying for a medical procedure that the patient may not remember. Keep information regarding what has been paid handy. If the patient or caregiver cannot remember the procedure or the person billing them, these documents will help you sort out problems.

Health care providers generally bill the patient for services while they are waiting for payment from the insurance company. It helped me to staple the billing from the doctor to the paid receipt from the insurance company once I had received both papers. At the end of the month, I would remove all of the "paid by insurance" forms and the "billed by health care providers" forms that matched and file them at home. I would call the insurance company regarding any left over billings that did not have a paid by insurance form and ask if the bill for the procedure had been filed with insurance by the doctor. Some months I would have only a couple of charges and other months I could have more than a hundred charges. It all depended on where Nathan was on his treatment plan. It will help relieve both patient and caregiver of unnecessary work and confusion if they keep on top of these items.

Medical insurance is something one must keep on top of at all times. It can be confusing because of the way the health care providers bill the patient and the insurance company. Before ever paying for something a physician, hospital, or other provider has billed the patient for, contact the patient's insurance company and find out what their co-pay amount is for that treatment. Many times the patient's insurance company has an arrangement with the health care provider to pay an agreed amount for a procedure, which is less than what the health care provider bills the patient. The patient will not owe the difference. The bill will be corrected once the insurance company has paid. In other words, 2 + 2 does not always = 4 when dealing with a medical provider or insurance company. If there is confusion or a problem over a bill, physicians and other health care providers have billing offices that the patient or caregiver can call for help. Billing department employees can let you know the status of the claim and can help the patient or caregiver set up payments, if needed.

It is important for a patient to talk to his insurance company to find out what will be covered. Ask the patient's health care provider to confirm coverage and what the patient's estimated expenses will be on all treatments **before** the procedure occurs. Pre-certification with the insurance company is often required, even if they have said that they will cover a certain procedure. Acquiring the pre-certification ensures that your insurance will cover the expense. Insurance companies will not cover some procedures or treatments at all. Sometimes, you must prove "medical necessity" (in other words, the treatment is medically required not just desired by the patient) before an insurance company will pay for a procedure. The patient's doctors are very familiar with this and their employees will help you complete the process.

Learn about the patient's prescription plan, if there is one. Some plans allow full payment for all medication received while an inpatient is in a hospital, but do not cover any pharmacy charges after discharge. Many prescription plans insist on the use of generic medications rather than brand name prescriptions, and they may pay more for them. For example, the patient's co-pay for a generic medication would cost $10.00. But if the patient or caregiver insists on a brand name medication, the patient could pay $200.00. This is important information their doctors need to know so they can prescribe medications that the patient's plan will pay for. Remember, however, there may be valid reasons why the patient's physician wants to use the brand name product. While generic medication is cheaper, doses and quality can vary widely. The physician has the patient's best interest in mind. Insurance companies are primarily concerned with cost. Please call the patient's insurance company for clarification and use the workbook page titled "Insurance Prescription Plan" to document the information.

Understanding the patient's insurance policy is essential. Knowing who to call, how it works, what their coverage is, and the process the patient and their health care providers must use to receive all the benefits available is the key to reducing both the patient's and caregiver's stress and undue financial burdens.

In the three-ring binder, create a notebook titled "Insurance". This notebook is the patient's active unpaid balance notebook, which will constantly change as treatment continues. This notebook, as previously discussed, is for all bills sent to the patient by providers and the insurance benefits payment forms that explain what has been paid or not and why. You can use this notebook to keep up with all of the patients billing needs. Once the patient receives an invoice from a medical provider the patient or caregiver can file it by date and by procedure while waiting for the patient's insurance company to respond with their explanation of benefits payment forms. Once the patient or caregiver has received both, the they can match the two and find out if a balance is due. Once the bill is paid, remove it from the notebook and store the bill and the insurance form in a file at home for future reference. It is important to keep these bills and statements. If questions arise later, they are the patient's documentation regarding what was paid and why. Insurance companies are like the IRS: it is up to an individual to prove whatever is being questioned.

Use your notebook dividers. Place dividers in your notebook and label the dividers. The following headings are some examples.

Doctors Visits: Filed by date of service

Hospital Visits: Filed by date of service

Other Providers: Filed by date of service. This covers laboratory charges, radiology charges and other services not directly received from the hospital or physician's office.

Insurance Benefits: You will receive an "explanation of benefits" statement from your insurance company once payment has been paid to the health care professional.

What We Owe: Co-payments due or what is due after insurance has paid.

Completed Invoice: An invoice is considered complete, once the insurance company has sent you a copy of their explanation of benefits statement which itemizes the amount of money insurance has paid the provider, money owed by the patient and the amount of money written off due to a contract agreement between the provider and insurance company. You may see a zero balance or a co-pay amount. Pay this to the provider by check. Record the amount paid by the patient on the explanation of benefits statement, the date of your payment and the check number. Once the insurance company has paid the invoice and you have paid any remaining amount owed, remove the information from your notebook, attach notes for future reference and file it in a safe place.

Active: The only papers you should have in this notebook are active, unpaid bills.

Action Pending Health Care Provider: At the end of the month, contact the health care provider and request a statement from them to match your insurance company explanation of benefits statement so you have the provider's invoice recording any payments they have received.

Action Pending Insurance: If you have a bill from a doctor but do not have an explanation of benefits from your insurance company, call your insurance company customer service department and ask them if they have received an invoice from the health care provider. If they have not, ask the insurance company to request an invoice from the health care provider so you can close this invoice.

Transportation Costs: This includes documentation of mileage to and from health care services, cab fares, public transportation costs, and parking fees, all of which can be used as a deduction on your taxes. The IRS will require documentation, so keep these receipts.

You can personalize this section to fit your needs by creating tabs that reflect your needs.

Medicare and Medicaid Benefits:
Your Safety Net for the Journey

Medicare and Medicaid benefits continue to change, but there are cancer benefits for those who qualify. Place a call to your local office and request an outline of benefits for cancer care. Your oncologist's office often can be very helpful explaining Medicare and Medicaid benefits to you. Ask the business manager or his or her assistant to explain how Medicare and Medicaid works and the process you and the medical provider must comply with to receive coverage. Another source for assistance is through the social workers at local hospitals; they are well versed on Medicare and Medicaid Benefits. Remember, the health care provider wants to be paid for services rendered and the office staff members can often assist you in confirming coverage and benefits or refer you to someone else who can help.

It is also important to request information regarding Medicare and Medicaid medication benefits. This information changes regularly, so it is best to check with your pharmacy and doctors' offices often, to make sure you are prescribed the best medication for your condition and that the medication is covered by the plan. Supplemental health insurance and prescription coverage is advisable to receive the best health care available.

Please refer to the Medicare and Medicaid website for the most up-to-date benefits information at http://www.socialsecurity.gov or call this Social Security phone number to ask your questions about cancer disability medication assistance: 1-800-772-1213. This office is open Monday to Friday, 7am to 7pm.

Short-term and Long-term Disability and Social Security

Some people are able to continue working through all or part of their treatment. For others, it is necessary to take time off to continue their treatment. The concern about this can be overwhelming, but it does not need to be. This is time for you to take another deep breath and move into another "new normal place." This may be a temporary place or an extended one. Many employers provide insurance policies that cover employees for short-term disabilities as well as long-term disabilities. Many smaller companies, however, do not have disability insurance. Check with the human resources department at your company to find out if this is a service your company provides. You must request information from your company so that you can complete the necessary forms to activate the plan, if you have one. The plans do not automatically activate with a phone call.

Your company representative can explain the company plan and give you the length of time for short-term plan benefits as well as long term plan benefits, if available. Your representative can provide the forms you must complete to activate your plans. You must follow your company guidelines and continue to update their records with doctor's reports and treatment plans. Some companies require their company physicians to see you and you may be required to complete follow-up appointments.

You also need to call your local Social Security office and set up a telephone interview appointment for disability services. Social Security can be activated in addition to your company plan or if your company does not have a disability insurance plan you can request only Social Security assistance. They will send you a packet in the mail for you to complete before a telephone interview appointment. Social Security personnel schedule these interviews by appointment as if you were going to an office, but the interview is completed over the phone. **You must be at your phone at the scheduled time to complete the interview.** If you miss this call, it can take as long as six weeks to reschedule your telephone appointment.

Once the telephone interview is complete, you will need to have your doctor complete the disability forms to submit to Social Security. Schedule an appointment with the person who called you for your phone interview. He or she will schedule a time to meet with you personally to review your paperwork. You must have all of your papers in order and signed by your health care professionals at the time of this appointment. Anything left incomplete will delay and possibly disqualify the processing of your Social Security disability insurance claim.

Social Security processed and accepted our claim on the first try by following their directions exactly as stated. Many people must reapply. My tips about completing this process are:

- respond to every question as accurately as you can;

- complete each form; and

- gather from your doctors, all signatures, letters, and other forms requested that describe your illness and disabilities.

This will save a great deal of time and allow you to receive your benefits more quickly while unemployed. If you need assistance to process your claim, many attorneys specialize in Social Security law and can help.

When calling to find out about benefits for short- or long-term disabilities as well as Social Security benefits, you must be prepared to tell your service representative the type of cancer you have been diagnosed with, its prognosis, and the short- and long-term treatment plans your doctor has outlined. Your workbook provides examples of questions asked.

Many companies require an employee to apply for Social Security benefits before applying for their disability plans. This means Social Security will pay you your allowed benefit and the company plan will pay the difference between what Social Security pays you and your current wages. Many short-term disability plans are gradually decreased over a few months. This means you will be given your current salary for a few weeks and, after a set date, you will receive a percentage decrease for a certain number of weeks, followed by another percentage decrease until a date when long-term disability and Social Security funds may become available. Knowing and understanding how your plans work can assist you with financial decisions. Every employer's plan is different and each person's needs are different. The best way to find out what your options are is simply to call your place of employment, the Social Security office, and your health care providers to ask for assistance.

If you do not have short- or long-term disability insurance through work, you may apply immediately for Social Security disability benefits. No payments from Social Security, however, are payable for partial disability or short-term disabilities. The "Official Definition" is found in the Social Security Act. Social Security disability benefits will cover a percentage of your wages. You also may receive benefits to assist you with your expenses.

Remember to ask for assistance and guidance from medical providers. Your health care providers may be able to direct you to social services departments within hospitals and to other government agencies for additional options. They are there to help you with these processes and are a wealth of knowledge.

Please refer to the Internet web sites for up to date Social Security information at www.socialsecurity.gov or www.ssa.gov,

Or phone (800) 772-1213

The Disability Interview section on the website is extremely valuable.

Online Application SSA-3368-BK Disability Report

There is also an "On-line Starter Kit" available to help you apply for benefits.

If you phone, explain that you want to apply by phone, not on-line, for the Disability Report. This phone line is open Monday to Friday 7am to 7pm.

Social Security Checklist Application for Disability Coverage

You will need this information to be able to complete the disability forms. Application is easier if you gather this information before sitting down to complete the forms.

Medical Information:

- Name, addresses and phone numbers of all doctors, hospitals and clinics,

- Patient ID numbers

- Dates seen

- Names of medicines you are taking

- Medical records in your possession

Other Required Information:

An original certified copy of your birth certificate;

- If born in another country, Proof of US Citizenship or legal residency

- If you are or were in the military, an original or certified copy of your military records or service discharge papers, (form DD214) for all periods

- If you worked last year, copies of your W-2 form from your last year's taxes;

- If you were self-employed last year, copies of your Schedules C and SE IRS1040 forms

- If you had Workers Compensation information, date of injury, claim number and proof of payment amounts

- Social Security for your spouse and minor children

- Checking and savings account numbers, Name, address, phone numbers of a person to contact if you are unavailable

- Kinds of jobs and dates you worked in the last 15 years before you became unable to work

- Check the Social Security web site to make sure you have the most up-to-date information

Financial Assistance—Government-Funded Programs

The Following programs can offer assistance in addition to, or in place of, private disability insurance benefits.

Hill-Burton Program

www.hrsa.gov/osp/dfcr
(800) 492-0359
Health Resources and Service Administration
U.S. Department of Health and Human Services
Call for eligibility and a list of Hill-Burton programs offering low cost or free medical care.

Community Assistance Programs

Community assistance programs can help with transportation to and from medical appointments, home health care, medical billing, insurance, Medicare, Medicaid, and Social Security programs, homemaker and chore-maintenance services, adult day care, home meal delivery, telephone contact with home bound people living alone, legal assistance, mental-health services, and case management. The Area Agencies on Aging are one example and can refer you to other programs. Referrals to these programs can also be found through hospital social services departments and local government agencies. The phone book and the Internet can be very helpful locating these services for you. I have listed those that I am familiar with.

Area Agencies on Aging

www.eldercare.gov
(800) 677-1116

For financial assistance, emergency food, childcare, legal services, transportation to medical care facilities, low-cost pharmaceutical programs and health insurance, home meal delivery, try these agencies:

National Action Partnership

www.communityactionpartnership.com
(202) 265-7546
Assistance with treatment and financial needs

United Way of America

www.unitedway.org
(703) 836-7100

Meals for homebound people, nationwide delivery service

www.nationalmealsonwheels.org
(319) 358-9362

Home Health Care and Hospice Information

The patient's condition may require more extensive care than the home caregiver easily can provide. While it may be difficult to accept this, it is important for the patient, the caregiver, and the family to use assistance when it is necessary. It is a very personal decision. The extra help can add to the patient's, the caregiver's, and the family's quality of life. There are many agencies that are available through your medical team and your insurance company that provide home health care, rides to and from treatments and assistance, and hospice care.

If you find you have a need, concern, or a problem with any part of your treatment plan, it is best to first speak to the nurses at your doctor's offices. They are a wealth of knowledge and can give you information to solve most problems. Many people need assistance with rides to treatment, appointments, and health care.

The nurses can give you the names and telephone numbers of people to contact and how to go about arranging a ride program in your area. Some cities have a medical necessity ride share program. You can find out about these programs through your local city and transportation departments. Also, check with social workers at your local hospital for additional information to assist you with your needs.

Home health care assistance is also available. Home health care assists the patient and family to manage the demands of often unfamiliar medical care at home. It helps keep the patient at home, avoid inpatient hospital care, uncomfortable travel to and from medical facilities, and allows for a more comfortable setting. Carefully evaluate available programs to be sure whatever program you choose meets your needs and provides the kind of medical care that makes you feel comfortable. Your doctor can recommend home health care agencies. Contact your insurance company to find out which agency is under contract with your health insurance. It is important for you to find out the details from your insurance company, as there are limitations to some plans for home health care.

Once the doctor prescribes home health care, insurance is then informed. You will receive a call from the agency explaining how this program works within your area and you can schedule an appointment to complete the necessary paperwork. This is the "intake interview." Appointment times vary from agency to agency, so ask how long the intake appointment will take. Ours lasted about three hours. The nurses complete the paperwork, you complete paperwork, and the nurse completes a physical exam, orders supplies, and sets a time for a visiting nurse to arrive at your home for care. Generally, patients require several visits per day from home health nurses.

If the journey with cancer is ending, the patient, family, and caregiver can choose whether it is best to have the patient at home or in a medical facility. Hospice care can be at home or in a nursing care facility. The term "hospice" describes a program to care for patients without the medical constraints that are found when one is an inpatient in a hospital. Some people enter hospice care, recover for a time, and go home. Most people use hospice care near the end of their lives. The hospice nurses are amazing people who help the patient and the family with all of their needs. Hospice can be set up like home health care, if the patient would rather stay at home. Some patients opt to move into a health care facility that provides hospice care because they feel more comfortable. It is different for everyone and there is no right or wrong choice.

Hospice is available to help the patient as well as the family move through the stages of illness, ease the dying process, and initiate the healing process when death occurs. In hospice, the patient's comfort is of prime importance. Hospice provides the comfort and security that allows the patient to die with dignity, without pain, and surrounded by family. Whatever your decision about care, always inform your doctor about your needs and do not hesitate to ask for assistance.

Suggestions for People Dealing with Cancer Who are Without Caregiver Assistance

Many people live alone and do not have caregivers on a daily basis. There are many assistance programs in most areas to help you make your appointments, meet your medical needs, and get help at home. Talk to your doctor and ask him or her for guidance. This will help you begin gathering information about programs that fit your needs. I would suggest calling your city or local transportation office for medical transportation assistance and special needs ride sharing. Churches often provide assistance with home maintenance, household needs, and people to assist you with your grocery shopping. Groups such as Meals on Wheels is a great organization for assistance with meals as well as providing volunteers to check on people to see if they need assistance in other ways.

Some grocery stores offer personal shopping and delivery for a very reasonable price and sometimes at no charge. Simply call your local grocery store's customer service department and ask them if they have a program to assist disabled people with their shopping needs as well as a delivery service.

Home health care is also an option and your insurance will often assist you with payment and referrals. Many people need assistance taking baths, getting up in the morning, meal preparation, house cleaning, and other personal needs. Home health care agencies have programs to assist disabled people. The services offered are provided at an hourly wage based on the care required.

Social service department personnel at a hospital or through a city or state agency will guide you and help arrange for assistance. Simply call those agencies in your area and ask. Explain your health needs and ask what programs are available. Many services are at a prorated price, depending on your needs and whether volunteers or skilled people offer the service. Always be clear when asking for what you need so people can provide the best services.

Legal Issues

It is always important to have your legal affairs in order, whether you are ill or not, but it is especially true when dealing with cancer. I found discussing and arranging our personal affairs, care for our children, pets, home, belongings, and finances through an attorney to be most useful and reassuring. When a person dies without a will, the estate is described as "in testate." This means the state gets to decide how your estate is handled and the process of probate (settling estate) can be significantly delayed. It also means any wishes you had regarding your estate are unknown and likely will not be carried out.

Fortunately, we had met with our attorney about six months before Nathan's illness was diagnosed. This meant we did not have to deal with this process while under the stress of dealing with cancer. Having your affairs in order simply means that you have a:

- will stating how you want your estate (what you possess) handled,

- living will to explain your medical wishes should you not be able to speak for yourself, and

- medical power of attorney that appoints another person to make medical decisions for you if you cannot make them.

- Do not resuscitate document, known as the DNR which is needed if taken by ambulance to the hospital

We also wrote a letter to our children telling them how much we loved them and wanted them to fulfill their dreams so that they would know how much we loved and respected them. Once the attorney completed these documents, we signed them, had them notarized, and placed them in our safe deposit box. Our attorney also kept a copy of them. I highly recommend that you provide a copy to whomever you have asked to be executor of your will so that a court order will not be required to open your safe deposit box.

Nathan did not want to remain on life support should his life reach a point where he could not return to health. His choice was understandable and it was up to him to decide. Hospitals require a copy of your medical power of attorney and living will at the time of admission. If that is not available, they have the patient complete a form outlining his or her wishes and have two people witness it. It is very difficult to complete a form like this in an emergency. It is much easier to complete these forms when you are healthy and thinking clearly.

At the time of Nathan's last admission, hospital employees asked for these forms. It was difficult to turn those papers over to them because at that point I knew Nathan would not come home. It was also a relief to know that Nathan's wishes would be met without me having to make choices that would have pushed my emotions to the limit.

After Nathan's death, I needed to go to probate court to settle Nathan's affairs. Having all of Nathan's papers in order made this process less painful. I urge you to look at legal matters, speak to an attorney, and make sure your affairs are in order. It is well worth the time, effort, and expense, and adds to your wellbeing. The "Legal" section in your workbook provides a framework to guide you in these matters.

Personal Issues

I found, as a caregiver for my husband, that I lost who I was as a person. Looking back on everything that happened, I would change the way I handled some things, but I dealt with most everything from the bottom of my heart and soul. I think when you are going though a life-threatening illness of your own or that of a loved one, it is important to discover who you are and how that affects your beliefs. It is then important to try to act according to those beliefs.

Nathan and I firmly believed in making memories. We, as a family made a commitment to make lasting memories during Nathan's illness. We all loved him and we will carry his memory with us the rest of our lives. We continued to grow and change and our experiences during this time certainly helped to make us the people we are. Life happens, sometimes without our control, but we have the opportunity to make our memories good or bad.

It was important for my family to share our closeness, as well as to live our dreams. While Nathan was ill, we lived for the moment because we knew our moments were few. Nathan died at 49 years of age—one daughter was in college and one was in high school. It was the day before her prom. I was 46 years old, and that day I became a widow with two children. Of course, this was not our plan, but it was what life brought to us. We had to rise and live without a husband and father.

I closed my business shortly after Nathan's diagnosis so I would have more time to care for him and our daughters, Kaela and Sorrell. This is not always possible for everyone; however, I wanted that time to be the best wife and mother I could be during our limited time together. Making this choice was one of the best choices I made. It gave us time to be a family and make memories for our daughters and for myself. We chose to reduce our expenses, live as frugally as possible, and enjoy each other. The house, the car, and the rest of our possessions were not what were important. They would be there when Nathan was gone, but the chance to be with him would no longer be available. If this is not possible for you, try to find a way to meet your needs in another way.

Nathan required round the clock medical care while at home. I chose to learn how to provide basic care such as changing dressings, cleaning his IV sites, and giving medications. I chose this because I did not want to have home health care nurses at our home at all hours. This choice offered us the freedom to relax together and take care of medical needs at our convenience. For example, I was able to change his dressing myself when he woke up rather than having to wake him up because a home health person had arrived and needed to complete the task. Home health professionals can provide training for this type of medical care. This removed the burden of scheduling this care, and gave us a sense of peace and freedom. Remember, you have to decide for yourself about this. Some people feel overwhelmed, frightened, or burdened by taking on this care. Don't feel as if you have let your family member down if you cannot provide this. There is excellent care provided by home health professionals and hospice staff. Use it if you need it.

As well as providing Nathan's medical care, I discovered that by becoming Nathan's nurse, I also became the person who brought him some physical pain from time to time. This turned me into his caregiver/nurse rather than Dianna his wife. As a result, we lost some closeness that we had shared in our relationship. It was almost as if I became his parent rather than his wife. I missed being Dianna and his wife when I become his caregiver and nurse. It was a difficult choice and a difficult job, but one I am glad I took on.

I found that keeping a journal helped me release emotions, discover feelings, and heal myself as we went through Nathan's illness and death. It is so important to write to yourself, speak to other people, read for pleasure, and find your comfortable place—whatever works for you. There were many times when Nathan would become angry, upset, or frightened while on his chemotherapy medications. He did not sleep for days on end due to medications. He would become angry with me and say things to me that were the medications or illness speaking, not him. I would become hurt, angry, and upset. Not wanting to argue or be angry with him at these times, I learned to sit down at my computer and just type whatever was going through my mind. Once finished, I would not re-read the words; I would simply press the delete key and flush those feelings away as if flushing a toilet. I did not hold onto the anger or frustration, I simply flushed it away with the delete key. This may or may not work for you. If not, it may be important for you to have someone—a friend or therapists—to talk to who will listen and help you deal with your feelings.

Nathan went through seven near-death experiences that caused us a great deal of pain, sadness, and fear each time. Writing on my computer about those experiences and deleting them helped me process what was happening without spreading my anxieties to others. A release of emotion is so important however you chose to accomplish it. There is no right or wrong way, unless it burdens or causes pain for another. Releasing is important and for me was a very powerful way to deal with negative emotions. You may discover, as I did, that energy builds within your body that you need to release in a positive way. I found puffing pillows around the house helped me deal with the physical energy that built while I sat at appointments and while driving and not being able to exercise. Fluffing pillows was a release of energy. I enjoyed the look of the pillows once puffed and as an added bonus, I found them inviting for a restful nap.

As caregivers, we assume responsibility for our loved one who is ill and we also must still care for our children. Unfortunately, when someone is seriously ill the list of needy people can grow to include our extended family, friends, neighbors, and co-workers. The list can become endless. I found a strength within me that helped me through each day for nearly six years. I am grateful for the many people who helped us. I felt their energy. It kept us going in a positive direction and enabled us to meet the needs of each day. If I looked at each day as a fresh beginning and focused on that day's events, it helped me live that day to its fullest. If I had looked at the days or weeks ahead when rising in the morning, I would not have been able to get up.

I urge you to rest. Take time for a walk, listen to your favorite music, and enjoy a meal with a friend so you remain yourself. I did find some relief for myself. When feeling very sad I would stop at a card shop and simply read the funny cards until I could smile or laugh. It helped me step out of the caregiver role and take care of myself. Humor is very important and helped me treat those around me in a more relaxed fashion. Our medical team also would joke with us to help us see a positive side. Family and friends needed that boost as well.

As caregivers, we receive all of the news (bad as well as good) from the medical team. We must relay this information to others. If I focused on the good things and gave people information in a positive way, I found they did not treat Nathan as if he was dying. I would receive test results that indicated his cancer was advancing quickly and he required more treatment. I explained this to family and friends by telling them Nathan's tests were outside of normal. I told them he will be going back on treatment and the treatment he would be receiving offered many chances for remission for an extended time. I explained that there would be some days that were challenging, but remission was around the corner. By giving that message to family and friends, he would receive cards, calls, and visitors. All of this gave him a positive attitude and helped him to enter yet another treatment phase. Cancer treatment is not fun and can cause suffering from extremely unpleasant side effects. If your loved one knows deep within that life is worth living, that attitude alone can help pull him or her through a difficult treatment.

E-mail was a great way for us to communicate with family and friends on a daily basis, helping them to stay informed. We received so many phone calls that we could not keep up with them. Phone calls can be exhausting (and expensive, if long distance) because each person wants to know the same information and the treatment plan. Repeating this can create a great deal of stress. E-mail keeps people informed and can be sent out each day as a bulk mailing with only a few lines to say hello to everyone and a brief description as to what is happening. This worked well for us and everyone was informed.

TIP

You may want to create a web site with a web log (BLOG). You as the caregiver can create this site, tell family and friends the web site address and update it daily. People can post notes and comments which can be read by the patient, caregiver, family and friends. It's a great way to communicate, send pictures and keep in touch. Many hospitals are placing computers in rooms for patients and families to use. Some hospitals have not updated their rooms but patients are welcome to bring a lap top computer in to the room and connect with the web. This can assist the patient and family with research as needed, communication, staying connected with the outside world, as well as relieves stress. Hospital stays can be long and anything that you can do to keep connected with the outside world will help pass the time.

It is difficult to keep lives normal when "normal" is far from the reality you've always known. It can become possible when you discover "A New Normal". This is a place where you feel comfortable and can find activities to do, places to go, and are able to enjoy each other. It is a place that offers enjoyment while offering us what we need medically, personally, and emotionally. Before cancer, our family skied, hiked, played soccer, went on vacations, and engaged in many other physical activities. Once cancer arrived, we rented movies, went for walks, and had friends and family visits instead. All of these brought us joy and kept us active, but in a different way that accommodated how we were able to live at that time.

Always focus on what you believe is important. This will bring you joy, and joy keeps you moving in the direction that serves you best. Remember, medical facilities have wonderful people available to assist you with any of your needs. We spoke to our doctors and nurses, hospital chaplains, social service people, patient advocates, therapists, hypnotherapists, and by taking advantage of what they offered we kept ourselves in a place that felt safe, informed, physically and emotionally cared for, well educated, and supported.

Looking back on our experience, our family learned many things while on this journey. Family and friends became very close and we discovered the true meaning of these relationships. The person with cancer truly travels that road on his or her own. Caregivers, family, and friends can only accompany the patient on their journey. The patient must face the threat of his or her possible death and experience the discomfort and pain. Nathan said that, at times, he had to be there alone. He had to decide how to fight to stay alive and when it was time to stop. The caregiver can support and care for the patient, as well as help find the best treatments, but the patient is the one who must decide when the time has come to call it finished. It is a very personal decision for the patient, and it is very important that caregivers, family, and friends accept the patient's decision.

Raising Successful Children

At the time of Nathan's diagnosis, our daughters were in junior high school and elementary school. It was a time when we came together as a family. Each of us had our talents that helped bring us together, kept our lives on track, and gave us a special place in each others' hearts. Each child is so different in the way he or she accepts life's lessons.

Kaela, our elder, was "the communicator". Kaela had experienced many illnesses throughout her life that required hospitalization. She feared hospitals and had a very difficult time walking into one. She wanted to help her father and visit with him, but it was difficult for her to do on a daily basis. Her solution was to write e-mail and send it out to our family and friends to keep everyone up to date with Nathan's progress. We were tired and needed rest, yet family and friends needed information about Nathan. It was stressful for them not knowing how things were going, and it was stressful for us to have to keep up. The short e-mail messages Kaela sent to people helped them keep in touch with us, feel as if they were part of our lives, and allowed them to share their love with us. It also reduced the strain for us. Many people responded to those e-mails, which we read to Nathan while he was resting.

Sorrell, our younger daughter, was "the caregiver". She kept things together at home and brought things to the hospital when she became old enough to drive. She was by her Daddy's side, doing homework, working on school projects, and being a kid. We had her 16th surprise birthday at the hospital with her Daddy, a few friends, and medical people. It was our only way of being together over her birthday, and it created a lasting memory.

Both of our daughters wanted to be a part of decisions about their Dad's medical care. We shared with them information about his illness and treatment plans, what we thought and medical professionals thought about the options and gave them a chance to state their opinions. They seemed empowered by this. They also had some wonderful thoughts and advice to offer. Sharing this kind of decision-making is helpful to some children and for others it can be a burden. It is important for you to know your own children and if needed, seek advice from professionals to determine what is right for your family. Each family has different beliefs, faith, needs, and ways of coping. A child's age is important to consider as well. The way we handled things and the choices we made were right for us. I also found counseling for stress and grieving to be extremely important from the day of diagnosis.

Our family, friends, teachers, and community pulled together and offered support to us in so many ways. Teachers stayed after school with our daughters to help them complete their homework and car pools were arranged to take our children to all of their activities. Family and friends came to stay with our children when we were at the hospital and offered support by caring for our home and us and helping with anything we needed. Our daughters felt well loved.

Since their father's death, Kaela completed her Bachelor's degree in Interdisciplinary Studies and has now completed a Master's of Education with an emphasis in Montessori Education. Kaela and Justin (childhood friend) married five years after Nathan's death. Sorrell has one more year of college before she graduates with a Bachelor's of Fine Arts degree in Studio Arts and Art History. Each of them misses her father beyond words but his message was strong and loving to them. He wanted them to go after their dreams, live life to its fullest, and become the best they could be. Many people, before they die, will write cards to their children and ask their spouse to give the card to the child at an appropriate time such as graduation from college, their wedding, the birth of their first child, etc., in order to share their feelings with the child at a special time.

Raising children is never easy. Your relationship with your children before an illness occurs has a huge effect on how a child deals with illness and death. A relationship built on trust and the ability to express emotions makes the experience easier. Family and friends joining together during a time of illness, offers a child a pillar of strength and security while finding "A New Normal" place in life. Support and love are what we all need. It can be challenging, as many different kinds of emotions are present at any given time.

Keeping household rules consistent as before the illness or death helps a child to feel safe. The best thing to do is to keep in touch with your children, be open to their feelings and needs, and be aware of what is happening to them. You may notice children acting out or misbehaving. Recognizing where the behavior is coming from helps ease parental angst. It is so easy to be overwhelmed with tasks and your own emotions when a loved one is seriously ill that you lose touch with your children. It is extremely important to work with psychologists, counselors, and medical professionals to make sure you have an outlet for your emotions and needs and that the needs of your children are being dealt with in a positive and healthy way too.

Death

A diagnosis of cancer has often meant a death sentence in the past, but death is not always the outcome now. Diagnosis is better now and many cancer treatments offer a great deal of success. Death, however, is still a possibility. Initial information regarding a patient's type of cancer can be overwhelming, and it is important not to take the estimates of outcome as gospel. The doctors told us that Nathan had eight to ten months to live after his initial diagnosis; however, Nathan survived his cancer nearly six years longer. When death seems inevitable, though, it helps to see if there is not a more positive way to view a situation. I prefer, for example, to think that death was Nathan's healing. Nathan had a good quality of life for a little over three years, and then suddenly his cancer came out of remission. This began the long process of double bone marrow transplants and his gradual decline. He never recovered from the multiple myeloma.

I never believed I would be comforted by Nathan's passing until we experienced his final stage of disease. During his illness, we worked with medical professionals to keep his quality of life as high as it could be as we tried to cure his disease. Nathan had tried all the treatments available to him when his body gave up. His quality of life deteriorated significantly, and he was suffering. Nathan, Kaela, Sorrell, Nathan's parents, and I talked. We told him if it was time for him to be relieved from his suffering, we were ready to let go. We wanted him to find peace and comfort again. We called his brothers and sisters, our extended family and special friends for them to say their good-byes. Nathan was unable to speak to everyone, but he heard every word. At the end, he sat up in bed and attempted to say "I love you," took his last breath, and moved into a place of healing. It was a sad, but beautiful moment to hear his attempted words of love for us as we shared ours with him. He left us and was without pain, without suffering, and he was gone. I believe he had moved into a better place, a place where he was healed and happy.

We left the hospital on a beautiful sunny morning. Family and friends took us back to our home in Arlington, Texas, where we had lived for 19 years. Other family members and friends came over to talk to us and help. Everything was a fog. We were exhausted from the last week. We rested until we received a call from the hospital asking us to make our arrangements for Nathan. The word "arrangements" was as jolting as when we had heard the word cancer for the first time. How do we make arrangements and what are they? We were so numb from the past week and Nathan's death, we hurt in every part of our being and now we needed to make meaningful arrangements for Nathan. It was a blessing to have a friend whose husband had passed away just one month before Nathan and she guided me through each step.

We talked about Nathan's wishes and how to follow them. A friend from our support group helped me choose a funeral home based on her research. She told me about the different kinds of services funeral homes offer and their usual charges. We began by calling a funeral home whose personnel invited us to come in to discuss arrangements. Nathan wanted to be cremated and he did not want a funeral. He wanted us to celebrate his life with family and friends. The funeral home personnel were very helpful. They explained their procedures and showed us the urns available to contain Nathan's ashes. We decided to purchase three containers that represented Nathan's life through gift stores rather than the funeral home urns. It is important to talk to your local funeral home to discuss regulations about how ashes must be contained. We chose three urns because we were celebrating Nathan's life in three locations. We lived in Texas and had many friends there, but also had family and friends in Colorado and Massachusetts. We decided to have three celebrations of life for Nathan in different states and left an urn in each state for those who loved him and needed a place to remember him. It was easier for us to have three celebrations and spend time with those we love in each state, than have one large celebration and ask family and friends to travel to Texas.

The funeral home personnel arranged with the hospital to collect Nathan's body from the hospital and transport him to the funeral home. They also made arrangements with Dallas to transport Nathan's body to our city, completed the death certificate, and arranged for copies of his death certificates to be sent to our home at a later date. Request at least 10 copies of the death certificate, as you will need these to complete insurance and probate forms. The funeral home personnel asked us to identify Nathan before his cremation. We were able to spend time with him in the chapel at the funeral home for as long as we wanted. Nathan was then prepared for cremation. We left the containers we had chosen to hold his ashes at the funeral home and about a week later Nathan's ashes were returned to us. The funeral home gave us a form that allowed us to transport his ashes out of state for his celebrations of life. It is a legal requirement that if a person's body or ashes are transported out of state a form must accompany their remains. The funeral home also helped us place a notice in the paper regarding Nathan's death.

Celebrating Nathan's Life

Our first celebration was at our home one month after Nathan's death. We prepared our home by hanging pictures of his life collected by his sister Leslie around our home, and fixed his favorite foods and drinks for guests. We prepared a video showing many of the activities Nathan enjoyed and played it on the TV for people to watch. We ordered tables and chairs from a rental company so we had seating in our back yard around the pool for guests to enjoy their dinner, friendship, and time to remember our time with Nathan.

We had more than 300 people at Nathan's celebration. People brought their favorite Mexican dish and I had the main course catered by his favorite Mexican restaurant. People talked, ate, and drank, for about an hour. We then asked everyone to gather in the back yard around the pool. Nathan's close friend, Frank, began by talking about Nathan and the kind of person he was. Kaela, Sorrell, and I spoke about Nathan as a Dad and Husband. Our friend Margie played the viola while we read the song "Swimming to the Other Side" as we lit a candle for each year of Nathan's life and floated them across the pool in foil pans. A dear friend of Nathan's said a prayer for him and many of Nathan's friends spoke about him. We ended our celebration following Nathan's wishes by remembering him with joy, not sadness. He wanted us to celebrate his life and to celebrate our lives and experiences. We enjoyed dessert and many of us stayed and talked for hours as we honored Nathan's transition.

Many people were concerned about not having a funeral for Nathan, and we reminded them of his wishes. His wishes were different, but they were his and what he wanted after his death. Many people told me I should have a funeral anyway, but I could not have a funeral and go against his wishes. Instead, we prepared all three celebrations of life in the places Nathan loved with those he loved. We asked people to bring to the celebration a picture or a memory they had written, and to leave them in the basket at the door. This was comforting for people and the notes were memories we could read afterwards, which helped us heal. We read the notes and we had pictures of family and friends doing something special with Nathan to look at. I treasure those messages and those pictures to this day.

Our second celebration was in Colorado at my sister Susan, husband Randy and their children Alex and Elliot's home. Susan's family and my parents Frank and Gwendolyn graciously made the preparations for our extended family and friends from Colorado. We were married in Colorado and lived in Colorado for many years before moving to Texas. We had a similar celebration to the one in Texas. Instead of floating candles in a pool, a garden was planted by my sister and her family in their yard in Nathan's memory. We enjoyed food and drinks, family and friends, and remembered Nathan. His dear friend Ron began by asking everyone to join together share their memories. We said a prayer, lit candles around Nathan's garden, and celebrated our lives with him. We displayed pictures of the activities we had enjoyed together in Colorado and the people with whom we shared those joys. We again enjoyed Nathan's favorite foods and desserts and many of us stayed and talked for hours. We placed the second urn of Nathan's ashes on a cliff just above a pond with the ski area in the distance at my cousin's elk ranch in Steamboat Springs, Colorado, a place he had loved dearly.

Our third celebration was in Annisquam, Massachusetts, next to the ocean where Nathan's family enjoyed the summers. Nathan's parents Garth and Shirley, brothers Jeffrey and Brad, sisters Deborah and Leslie, sister-in-law Maureen, nieces Kelly, Emily, Warren, nephew Alex and friend John planned their celebration for family and friends gathered to enjoy a meal and to remember Nathan. We shared pictures of Nathan's life with one another, enjoyed our meal, and talked on the porch where we had always loved to gather to watch the sunsets over the water. After dinner we walked to his brother Jeffrey, wife Maureen, daughters Kelly and Emily's home nearby to share additional memories, then across to the beach where many guests kayaked out into the ocean to release a flaming watermelon at sunset. Nathan's family loved rivers, oceans and enjoyed kayaking, river rafting, and research of the Grand Canyon. The release of a flaming watermelon was symbolic of releasing a soul to forever float the waters. Nathan's brother, Brad, sang from a perch on the rocks jutting out from the ocean. Those of us on shore listened to his song and watched the sunset and the kayakers. We returned to the porch to enjoy dessert, and each other's company as we shared more memories of Nathan at the last of Nathan's celebrations. Nathan had been released from his life here, and those of us left behind must go through the grieving process in our own way. We must each find yet another "New Normal" place.

It is so important to pay attention and honor your wishes when a loved one dies, not what the world tells us to do. Our celebrations of life spoke to us in a very personal way. It was not what everyone might have done, but it was what was important to us. Many have told me since our celebrations that they have changed their last wishes to reflect our kind of celebration. It felt much more personal to them and it felt good to share in our lives. The celebrations were a time of complete togetherness, all in Nathan's memory. We remember him, love him, and will always cherish him in our hearts. Remember, do what is right for you. These memories will help bring you to a place of peace and harmony while processing your grief.

Not all cancers end in death, but I hope our experience helps you survive your experience with cancer. We bless all of you on your journey through cancer and healing.

Creating A Lasting Memory

Nathan was our daughters' soccer coach for nearly 15 years. He loved coaching kids and soccer. His dream was to set up a program where every child had the financial support to belong to a team, play soccer, exercise, and be a part of a bigger community. After Nathan's death, our family set up a fund called the Nate Marston Fund. In conjunction with the Colorado Rush Soccer Club, we arranged to raise funds to pay soccer registration fees for disadvantaged children and thus offer them an opportunity to play soccer. The fund now helps many children each year to be able to continue playing soccer or to begin playing soccer on developmental league teams.

Interested parties can visit our web site www.NateMarstonFund.com or visit the Colorado Rush Site at www.coloradorush.com. Those interested in donating can click on "donate" and share with the kids any amount they feel comfortable donating. All contributions are tax deductible. We also set up online shopping through Shop4Zero.com, which contributes 4% of all purchases to The Nate Marston Fund. Those interested in contributing to this fund can find an invitation on our web site at www.NateMarstonFund.com and click on the invitation to enroll.

Helping children play soccer in Nathan's memory has helped our family heal. It feels wonderful to assist children with their registration fees and to pay for "extras" that parents may not be able to afford. In this way, we feel Nathan's dreams are alive and being fulfilled. We honor his memory, remember him in a positive way, help others, and feel at peace. We greatly appreciate all contributions, and, through volunteer help, nearly 100% of the funds raised reach the children.

I encourage you to look at something special your loved one has enjoyed, believed in, or been a part of during their lives and find a way to keep this memory alive. It is healing to help others. This positive contact with people allows you to remember your loved one, talk about your experiences, and process your grief.

Workbook: After Diagnosis and the First Few Medical Appointments

This section of your workbook will assist you with documenting information needed after diagnosis and the first few medical appointments.

Doctor's Name: _____

Phone Number: _____

Fax: _____

After Hours Emergency Number: _____

Email: _____

Contact Person, Nurse, Medical Assistant, In case the doctor is unavailable:

_____

_____

_____

Your team of doctor's names and telephone numbers:

_____

_____

_____

_____

_____

_____

_____

_____

_____

Name of Hospital: _____

Phone Number: _____

Fax Number: _____

Contact Person: _____

Contact Person's Phone Number: _____

Fax Number: _____

Email: _____

Directions to the Hospital:

_____

_____

_____

_____

_____

_____

Date of diagnosis:

_____

_____

What type of cancer has been diagnosed?

_____

_____

_____

_____

_____

_____

_____

Stage of cancer (Stage 1, early stage cancer—Stage 4, late stage cancer) and what determines the staging of this cancer?

_____

_____

_____

_____

_____

Date and description of first symptoms:

_____

_____

_____

_____

_____

_____

_____

Describe how you feel right now (fatigue, pain, discomfort, pain scale: 1–10)

_____

_____

_____

_____

_____

_____

_____

_____

What is my prognosis (what you can expect while going through your treatment and long term quality of life)?

_____

_____

_____

_____

_____

Explanation of treatment plan:

_____

_____

_____

_____

_____

_____

Suggested research information about my type of cancer and where I can go to obtain this information (books, Internet sites, libraries, research libraries in hospitals for doctors and patients?

_____

_____

_____

_____

_____

_____

_____

_____

What is the best and healthiest approach to dealing with my cancer and what are my options?

_____

_____

_____

_____

_____

_____

_____

_____

_____

What tests have been done so far and what are the results?

_____

_____

_____

_____

_____

_____

_____

_____

_____

Please explain what these test results mean. Which results would indicate an improvement in my health and which results would indicate that I am not doing well?

_____
_____
_____
_____
_____
_____
_____

Please describe where we go from here:

_____
_____
_____
_____
_____
_____
_____
_____
_____
_____
_____

Record possible treatment options for your form of cancer. Place a "C" for conventional medicine (standard medical care), "CM" for complementary medicine (care with herbs, hypnotherapy, dietary supplements, etc.) "A" for alternative options (a treatment plan which does not include standard care but is made up of herbal, supplement to diet, etc.) next to suggested treatment options.

_____
_____
_____
_____
_____
_____
_____
_____

List how treatments and medications will affect your life: Side effects, and changes you may feel and the reason for those of prescribed medications, dosages.

_____
_____
_____
_____
_____
_____
_____
_____
_____
_____
_____

If I want to postpone the treatment recommended until I have had a chance to do some research how much time do I have before we need to take action?

_____
_____
_____
_____
_____
_____
_____
_____

What does my insurance plan cover?

_____
_____
_____
_____
_____
_____
_____
_____

Are there assistance programs within the hospitals, your office, or social services I might contact to help my family with our needs (lodging, travel) while I am being treated?

_____

_____

_____

_____

_____

_____

_____

_____

Notes:

_____

_____

_____

_____

_____

_____

_____

_____

_____

_____

_____

_____

_____

_____

_____

_____

_____

_____

_____

_____

_____

_____

Medical Insurance Coverage for the Cancer Patient

Who is your Medical Insurance Company?

_____
_____
_____

Do you have more than one insurance company? If so, keep things separate for each insurance company and create tabs following the same procedure as with insurance company number one and place it in your three ring binder following the same instruction for your notebook:

Does the insurance company have a person within the claims department I can work with on a regular basis, possibly a caseworker?

Name: _____Phone #: _____

Fax #: _____ Email: _____

Mailing address: _____

Your representative: _____

Policy number: _____ Group number: _____

Additional information on your card you may need for future reference:

_____
_____
_____
_____
_____
_____
_____
_____

Remember to write down the date, time, and person you spoke to when contacting the insurance company should you have additional questions.

Do I have cancer treatment coverage?_____

How much coverage?

_____

_____

_____

How does my cancer insurance coverage work? What are my limitations?

_____

_____

_____

_____

_____

_____

_____

_____

_____

_____

_____

_____

_____

_____

_____

_____

What are my co-pays for medical providers? Is this co-pay different for doctor's appointments, medical procedures, or testing?

_____

_____

_____

_____

Do I have a medical deductible to meet before coverage begins?

_____

_____

_____

_____

What is my yearly deductible? (Is it calendar year or does it begin in the middle of the year and ends in the middle of the year?)

_____

_____

_____

_____

Do I need a referral before seeing a medical professional?

_____

_____

_____

_____

Do I have a cap on my insurance plan? (Example: Some insurance plans will only cover $250,000 for lifetime claims and will not cover any claims above that)

_____

_____

_____

_____

_____

What kind of coverage do I have for medications? Some plans allow full payment for all medication given while as an inpatient in a hospital, but do not cover outpatient medications. Many prescription plans pay more for generic medications than for brand name products. This is something you need to know so you can inform your doctor and the correct medication can be prescribed and be covered by your insurance plan.

_____

_____

_____

_____

_____

Should you file for medical reimbursements or will your claims be filled directly by the pharmacy:

_____
_____
_____
_____
_____
_____
_____
_____
_____
_____
_____
_____
_____

Length of time to receive reimbursements:

_____
_____
_____
_____
_____
_____
_____
_____

Coverage for clinical trials:

_____
_____
_____
_____
_____
_____
_____
_____

Does the insurance company have a patient advocate to assist you with any needs you have now or may have in the future.

_____

_____

_____

_____

_____

_____

_____

_____

_____

_____

_____

_____

_____

_____

_____

_____

_____

_____

_____

_____

_____

_____

_____

_____

_____

_____

_____

_____

_____

_____

_____

_____

Medications

Many medications treat cancer, and this is known as chemotherapy. All medications have side effects and you need to be aware of these as well as the interaction these drugs may have with medications you currently take. Chemotherapy is a way to control the growth of or kill cancer cells and to try to place the patient into a remission (absence of cancer cells). Many of these medications can affect your balance, your ability to drive, drink alcohol, and take other medications; some of these drugs also can affect your personality. It is important for you to make a list of all medications you are taking, the dosage, what the medication is used for, the date you began taking the medication, and the date of completion. This will help you and your health care practitioners keep track of things.

It is also very important to inform your doctors about any supplement, energy drink, herb, or vitamins you take, as well as anything (other than food) that enters your body or that you apply to your skin. Many chemotherapy medications are drugs taken to control the growth or kill cancer cells, but chemotherapy doses are so high that anything else you take or use can interfere with treatment or cause unanticipated adverse effects.

Prescription Plan

Name of your **Prescription Plan:** _____
Address:

_____
_____
_____

Phone: _____ Fax: _____
Email: _____
Your representative: _____
Policy number: _____ Group number: _____
Additional information on your card you may need for future reference:

_____
_____
_____
_____

Name or your **Primary Pharmacy:** _____
Phone #_____Fax #_____
Email: _____
Mailing address:

_____
_____
_____
_____
_____
_____

Prescriptions filled by this pharmacy:

Doctor	Treats	Date	Rx #

You may need to use your own pharmacy as well as hospital pharmacies and mail-in pharmacies required by your insurance plan. The additional space below is for this information.

Hospital Pharmacy Name: _____

Address:

_____

_____

_____

Phone: _____ Fax: _____

Email: _____

Prescriptions filled at this pharmacy:

Doctor	Treats	Date	Rx #

Mail-In Pharmacy Name_____

Phone # _____Fax #_____

Email: _____

Mailing address : _____

Prescriptions filled by this pharmacy:

Date	Rx #	Doctor	Treats

<u>Additional Pharmacy</u> Name_____

Phone #_____Fax #_____

Email: _____

Mailing address: _____

_____

_____

Prescriptions filled by this pharmacy:

Date	Rx #	Doctor	Treats

<u>Additional Pharmacy</u> Name_____

Phone #_____Fax #_____

Email: _____

Mailing address: _____

_____

_____

Prescriptions filled by this pharmacy:

Date	Rx #	Doctor	Treats

Summary of All Prescriptions Prescribed By A Doctor

Rx #/name   dosage/times   Reason for taking   Start/Finish Pharmacy

_____
_____
_____
_____
_____
_____
_____
_____
_____
_____
_____
_____
_____
_____
_____
_____
_____
_____
_____
_____
_____
_____

All Products Applied to Your Skin

Products   Reason for taking   Start/Finish

_____

_____

_____

_____

_____

_____

_____

_____

_____

_____

_____

_____

_____

_____

_____

_____

_____

_____

_____

_____

_____

_____

All Supplements Taken Internally, Herbal Support And Drinks or Pills Taken

Name	Dosage	Reason for taking	Start/Finish

Vitamins

Name	Dosage	Reason for taking	Start/Finish

Side Effects

Please keep a copy of side effects your drug may cause in this folder and make notes here:

_____
_____
_____
_____
_____
_____
_____
_____
_____
_____
_____
_____
_____
_____
_____
_____
_____
_____
_____
_____
_____
_____
_____
_____
_____
_____

Short-term, Long-term Disability and Social Security

When calling to find out about benefits for short-term or long-term disability from your employer as well as Social Security benefits, you must be prepared to tell the service representative the type of cancer you have been diagnosed with, its prognosis, and the short-term and long-term treatment plans. They can explain the plans available to you, clarify the length of time for each plan, your benefits and explain what you must complete to activate your plan. You must follow their guidelines and continue to update their records with medical reports and treatment plans. Many companies require a patient to apply for Social Security benefits first. This means Social Security will pay you your allowed benefit and the company plan will pick up the difference. If you do not have short- or long-term disability insurance through work, you can apply for Social Security disability. Social Security disability typically covers an allowed amount that often is less than your current wages.

Your company's human resources telephone number: _____

Your representative: _____

Phone #_____Fax#: _____

Email: _____

Mailing address: _____

_____

_____

_____

_____

_____

_____

_____

Local Social Security office and contact person
Name: _____
Phone #_____Fax # _____
Email: _____
Mailing address: _____
_____
_____

Be prepared to give the Social Security number of the patient. Keep this Social Security number in a safe place to protect you from identity theft.
Time for your Social Security appointments: _____
Phone appointment time: _____
Be sure you are at your phone a few minutes early with your <u>ENTIRE</u> packet completed and <u>SIGNED BY ALL DOCTORS</u>.
Office appointment time: _____
Address for appointment: _____
<u>Arrive about 15 minutes early for your appointment with your entire packet completed and again, signed by all doctors</u>.

Legal

Attorney's Name: _____
Phone # _____ Fax # _____
Email: _____ Mailing Address: _____
_____
_____

Date completed: _____
Safe place to find legal documents _____
_____
_____
_____
_____
_____

Who else has a copy of these documents?
_____
_____
_____
_____
_____
_____
_____
_____
_____
_____
_____

You will reach your "New Normal."

Your dreams, reality, and life will change because of this experience.

Give yourselves space to grow and accept.

Never forget.

Always treasure the memories dear to your heart and soul.

They are yours to treasure for life!

Dianna Mitchell Marston

Contact Information

Dianna Mitchell Marston

P.O. Box 280176

Lakewood, CO 80228-0176

Email: Dianna Marston@anewnormal.com

www.anewnormal.com

Index

978-0-595-44899-9
0-595-44899-2